Back to Basics
5-Week Restart

Notice: This book is is not intended to replace recommendations or advice from physicians or other healthcare providers. Rather, it is intended to help you make informed decisions about your health and to cooperate with your healthcare provider in a joint quest for optimal wellness. If you suspect you have a medical problem, I urge you to seek medical attention from a competent medical provider.

Andrea Pouncy Waite

Garden of Wellness

1172 W. Galbraith Road

Cincinnati, Ohio 45231

HTTP:// www.garden-wellness.com

HTTP://www.andreawaitewellness.com

Back to Basics 5-Week Restart

ISBN-13: 978-1540757814

ISBN-10: 1540757811

This book is dedicated to leading others from all over the world to live healthier and safe lives. Through wellness, peace and happiness, to spread a message of health and well-being.

Contents

INTRODUCTION... 6

AWAKE.. 9

BALANCE 12

DISCOVER 27

RESET 42

GROWTH 45

Introduction

Food and its purpose has been in a constant evolution over centuries. Food once was looked upon as a key fundamental to life and medicine to cure and heal our bodies. Many foods and species have been used historically as remedies. Such as ginger to aid in digestion and treat nausea. Honey used by Egyptians to treat wounds. Greeks ate onions for their curative qualities and Romans used garlic for strength and immunity boosting effects. Moringa has been used in India's ancient traditions as a powerful health enhancing plant, as an excellent source of nutrition and energy booster. Indians and Mayans was a major group that used various herbal remedies from nature.

Fast forward into today, the things we eat now are not the same. What happened? Why have we lost our intent to eat and our relationship with food. We once possessed a relationship with nature and established a connection with food. While using a holistic approach to empathize disease prevention through one's pursuit of mental, physical, and emotional harmony with the environment. The beauty of food as medicine is that the choice to heal and promote health can begin as soon as your next meal.

Which is why being in school for Massage Therapy opened my eyes to natural ways of treating the body. I became fascinated with the science of alternative and complementary practices. Being balanced as a whole I wanted to learn and explore more. After I learned the benefits of living a holistic lifestyle I incorporated all aspect of holistic approaches to my life, quickly realizing its overall benefits. I also had struggled with acne and hyper-pigmentation which spark my interest in becoming a skin therapist/esthetician. Other than Massage Therapy and Esthetics I became interested in other forms of alternative healing from energy work, aromatherapy, holistic skincare and nutrition. I came to the realization that massage, skin, and nutrition are closely connected with physical emotional health, all being largely dependent on the mind, body, and spirit. All of which aids in creating optimal health and balance throughout for pure organic healing.

Treating my body naturally and holistically was a lifestyle change that created my strong interest in nutrition. I have been eating clean since August 1, 2013, transitioning to Vegan February 1, 2014, and went to mostly Vegetarian diet since March 1, 2014. I transformed my body and health, I weighed 278 lbs. I got down to 169 lbs, continued my goals and reached 156lbs. Loosing a total of 122 lbs. All achieved with pure organic healing through food. going back to the basics. When food was simple... Without shakes, pills, supplements, avoiding foods which are processed or been degraded of their nutritional quality, and eating home-cooked meals created in your kitchen. But, most importantly being able to know where your foods come from and how it is prepared.

The importance of proper digestion is well known to most health conscious people. Hippocrates (460-370 BC), the father of modern medicine, said "disease starts in the gut." But what fewer people realize is that while disease may start in the gut, it can advance all the way to the brain. For the most part, the body-mind connection has been explored in terms of how the mind, or our thoughts, impacts the body. This perspective comes from people who tend to live in their heads, believing that their bodies are somehow separate, lesser entities that need to be told what to do.

Having a healthy gut is crucially important for your overall well-being to obtain a balanced mood and energy levels, to have an optimistic outlook and to fully experience the joy of being alive. High quality, organic food is growing in popularity. We all know the devastating consequences of eating junk food and how important it is to eat healthy foods. To create a healthy digestive system, eat high quality, fresh foods that are prepared for easy digestion and absorption... EATING SIMPLE and with a PURPOSE.

With nutrition you can train yourself to get in touch with your own personal nutritional needs. You have to come from your gut! And the healthier your gut is, the easier it is to get in touch with it. My views in nutrition and wellness deals with the physical and mental health to achieve a positive 'mind body' relationship. This guide will be your foundation and blueprint in helping you change your eating habits and go back to eating with purpose.

How to use this book to reconnect with food and change your eating habits:

You will use this book as a guide to better engage you into going back to the basics of nutrition being looked at as a needed asset in health and healing.

By focusing on 5 components of change.

Learning from each step to make a lasting lifestyle change.

Week 1. Awake (precontemplation)

Week 2. Balance (contemplation)

Week 3. Discover (preperation)

Week. 4 Reset (action)

Week 5. Growth (maintenance)

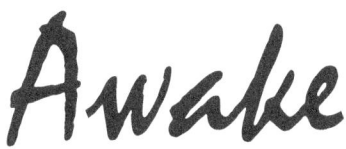

Awake

(contemplation) – "Problem Identified"

The first step to reconnect with food is to identify your problem with eating, by becoming fully aware of the nourishment available through the process of food preparation and consumption. You become aware of food and the eating process. Mindful eating is a practice that develops your awareness of eating habits and allows you to pause between your triggers and your actions. You can then change the emotional habits that have sabotaged your diet in the past. Mindfulness is paying attention to a particular way. Paying attention to purpose, in the present moment, and non judgmentally. Its self regulation of attention with an attitude, of openness, curiosity and acceptance.

Have you ever been connected to a certain taste or smell, and that taste or smell reminds you of a person in your life or a special moment in your life? For instance when I smell the scent of old spice I instantly connect that scent to my dad that passed away. Or when I taste a cherry pie I immediately think of my Grandma's cherry pies she used to make for my mom when she was alive. This is a form of connecting with food. We have more memories of smells, more memories of food sharing, more memories of flavors. Food connects us to memories that never fade. Which is being mindful when you eat plays a great importance in changing your eating habits.

Mindfulness is a technique for slowing down our lives and learning to live in the moment rather than obsessing about the past or worrying about the future. Its a way to relax and distance ourselves from the stressful and distressing thoughts. It's a practice based on Buddhist tradition in which our attention is focused on sensations in the present moment, without judgment, as a technique to quiet the mind. The techniques of mindfulness can be used with food, known as mindful-eating or conscious eating.

Principles of Mindful-Eating
- Chew, Chew, Chew. Each mouthful 35 times. Releases digestive enzymes, improves digestion and assimilation and satiety.

- Eat only when hungry. Do you really need a snack? Or is it a walk, a tall glass of water, or a rest that you truly require? Eat simple, whole foods. If it won't rot, don't eat it.

- Enough said! Drink Water. Chronic dehydration can cause fluid retention and bloating. You wouldn't wash your floors with milk or juice, would you? Water is the universal cleanser.

- Breathe, Relax, Feel. Use mealtime to connect with your body.

- Practice Gratitude. When we consciously and deeply acknowledge what we receive, we assimilate the benefits and open ourselves to the sense of abundance that we crave.

- Keep a food journal. Observe your body's responses to food and learn the truth of what works for you. Your needs may change with the seasons, stress levels and aging.

- Exercise every day. Whether it's yoga, walking, aerobics or swimming, daily exercise creates a healthy appetite. It also tones all our muscles and organs, oxygenates our brain and creates feel good hormones. It is essential to good health.

Mindful eating is a way of connecting with and appreciating food as nourishment.

<u>Try this:</u>
•Eat in silence.
•Focus on the sight, the taste and the smell of the food before putting it into your mouth.
•Once in your mouth, notice the texture, the flavor, and any thoughts you are having as you chew.
•Consider the food's journey: from seed, to harvest, to market, to skillet, and so on.
•After you finish, note any sensations, such as satiety, wanting more, or digestive discomfort, etc.
•Remember to breathe throughout this exercise!

BREATHE:
Before you even pick up the food to eat, take a couple of deep breaths. In through the nose and out through the mouth. Just allow the body and mind settle.

NOTICE:
In addition to the physical senses, notice how the mind responds to the food. For example is the food met with displeasure in your mind?

FOCUS:
As you move the food towards your mouth, shift the focus away from the hands and more towards the eyes, nose and mouth. How does the food smell? What does it look like close up?

<u>Since most people eat for reasons other than physical hunger, the first question of:</u>

- **"Why do I eat?"** is often central to ultimately changing behavior.

- **"Why do I eat?"** may include an exploration of triggers such as physical hunger, challenging situations, or visual cues, which often spring from stress, fatigue, or boredom.

- **"When do I want to eat?"** The answer may depend on the clock, physical hunger cues, or emotions.

- **"What do I eat?"** examines the factors people consider when choosing food, such as convenience, taste, comfort, and nutrition.

- **"How do I eat?"** Is eating rushed, mindful, distracted, or secretive? In our technological, on-the-go society, exploring the process of eating can be eye-opening.

- **"How much do I eat?"** Quantity may be decided by physical fullness cues, package size, or habit.

- **"Where does the energy go?"** Eating may be invigorating, cause sluggishness, or lead to guilt and shame. How is the energy used during work or play?

It is also important to look at all the foods and ingredients you are eating rather than focus on just one. If not, you may inadvertently limit your access to quality foods and drinks. For instance, high fructose corn syrup is often mislabeled as "bad," even though there is no credible scientific evidence to support this claim. Instead, look at all of the combined sugars in your diet and make healthy decisions accordingly.

Be aware of what you are eating and its nutritional value. What amounts of calories, fat and carbohydrates are in the foods you eat? Read labels and become food-conscious to make healthy eating decisions.

Balance

(contemplation) – "Motivated To Change"

In today's fast-paced, high-demand world, we have become a culture focused on convenience and that includes how we eat. Many might find that preparing a fresh cooked meal impossible on a daily bases. With the epidemic rise of obesity and diabetes, the link to your health and what you eat has taken control over our lives. Which is why what you eat determines your overall health. The first step is gaining your intent of eating is to find balance. The saying goes when you find balance start with a mindset shift and willingness to let go and enjoy life. Healthy eating starts with the right attitude. First remembering the importance of food is to fuel and nourish the body. Learn to reconnect with food again. Stop looking at food as choir and something that is non enjoyable. Do not let eating healthy consume your emotional thoughts by over analyzing what you are consuming and when to consume.

Now that you are aware and you have identified the problem, begin to cultivate balance. Create a healthy relationship between your thoughts. It is often said the if you can not control your thoughts you can not control your behavior. Self discipline begins with the mastery of your thoughts. Gain the willpower to train your mind and the body will follow.

Many people may say they cant find time. What do you do if you want to eat healthier, but you don't have time to cook, and your lack of energy, causes you to cave into to junk food?

The answer is simple. Let's examine how you spend your time, and whether you are making the most of it. Try to organize each day according to the priority level of tasks to be accomplished. Without priorities to guide your decisions, your calendar will be overrun with responsibilities that don't fulfill your life or help you reach your goals. If you have a plan mapped out to the goals you want to achieve you will be more motivated to implement those goals. When you see your goals laid out in front of you, you will become more motivated to change.

Make your record fairly detailed. For example: 8:00 – 9:00 worked out, 9:30 - 10:00 watched television. Try to record your activities as you go. If you try to record them all at once at the end of the day, or even worse, at the end of the week, you will not be able to remember what you did. By doing this will see what takes up most of your time and what you are allowing to interfere with incorporating healthy eating into your life.

DAY ONE

Time	Planned Activity	What I actually did...
Example	**Work out**	**Went to a party**
5:00 am		
5:30 am		
6:00 am		
6:30 am		
7:00 am		
7:30 am		
8:00 am		
8:30 am		
9:00 am		
9:30 am		
10:00 am		
10:30 am		
11:00 am		
11:30 am		
12:00 noon		
12:30 pm		
1:00 pm		
2:00 pm		
2:30 pm		
3:00 pm		
3:30 pm		
4:00 pm		
4:30 pm		
5:00 pm		
5:30 pm		
6:00 pm		
6:30 pm		
7:00 pm		
7:30 pm		

8:00 pm		
8:30 pm		
9:00 pm		
9:30 pm		
10:00 pm		
10:30 pm		
11:00 pm		
11:30 pm		
12:00 am		

DAY TWO

Date: ____/____/_____

Time	Planned Activity	What I actually did...
Example	**Work out**	**Went to a party**
5:00 am		
5:30 am		
6:00 am		
6:30 am		
7:00 am		
7:30 am		
8:00 am		
8:30 am		
9:00 am		
9:30 am		
10:00 am		
10:30 am		
11:00 am		
11:30 am		
12:00 noon		
12:30 pm		
1:00 pm		
2:00 pm		
2:30 pm		
3:00 pm		
3:30 pm		
4:00 pm		
4:30 pm		
5:00 pm		
5:30 pm		
6:00 pm		
6:30 pm		
7:00 pm		
7:30 pm		
8:00 pm		

8:30 pm		
9:00 pm		
9:30 pm		
10:00 pm		
10:30 pm		
11:00 pm		
11:30 pm		
12:00 am		

DAY THREE

Time	Planned Activity	What I actually did...
Example	**Work out**	**Went to a party**
5:00 am		
5:30 am		
6:00 am		
6:30 am		
7:00 am		
7:30 am		
8:00 am		
8:30 am		
9:00 am		
9:30 am		
10:00 am		
10:30 am		
11:00 am		
11:30 am		
12:00 noon		
12:30 pm		
1:00 pm		
2:00 pm		
2:30 pm		
3:00 pm		
3:30 pm		
4:00 pm		
4:30 pm		
5:00 pm		
5:30 pm		
6:00 pm		
6:30 pm		
7:00 pm		
7:30 pm		
8:00 pm		

8:30 pm		
9:00 pm		
9:30 pm		
10:00 pm		
10:30 pm		
11:00 pm		
11:30 pm		
12:00 am		

DAY FOUR

Date: _____/_____/ _____

Time	Planned Activity	What I actually did...
Example	**Work out**	**Went to a party**
5:00 am		
5:30 am		
6:00 am		
6:30 am		
7:00 am		
7:30 am		
8:00 am		
8:30 am		
9:00 am		
9:30 am		
10:00 am		
10:30 am		
11:00 am		
11:30 am		
12:00 noon		
12:30 pm		
1:00 pm		
2:00 pm		
2:30 pm		
3:00 pm		
3:30 pm		
4:00 pm		
4:30 pm		
5:00 pm		
5:30 pm		
6:00 pm		
6:30 pm		
7:00 pm		
7:30 pm		
8:00 pm		

8:30 pm		
9:00 pm		
9:30 pm		
10:00 pm		
10:30 pm		
11:00 pm		
11:30 pm		
12:00 am		

DAY FIVE

Date: _____/_____/ _____

Time	Planned Activity	What I actually did...
Example	**Work out**	**Went to a party**
5:00 am		
5:30 am		
6:00 am		
6:30 am		
7:00 am		
7:30 am		
8:00 am		
8:30 am		
9:00 am		
9:30 am		
10:00 am		
10:30 am		
11:00 am		
11:30 am		
12:00 noon		
12:30 pm		
1:00 pm		
2:00 pm		
2:30 pm		
3:00 pm		
3:30 pm		
4:00 pm		
4:30 pm		
5:00 pm		
5:30 pm		
6:00 pm		
6:30 pm		
7:00 pm		
7:30 pm		
8:00 pm		

8:30 pm		
9:00 pm		
9:30 pm		
10:00 pm		
10:30 pm		
11:00 pm		
11:30 pm		
12:00 am		

DAY SIX

Time	Planned Activity	What I actually did...
Example	**Work out**	**Went to a party**
5:00 am		
5:30 am		
6:00 am		
6:30 am		
7:00 am		
7:30 am		
8:00 am		
8:30 am		
9:00 am		
9:30 am		
10:00 am		
10:30 am		
11:00 am		
11:30 am		
12:00 noon		
12:30 pm		
1:00 pm		
2:00 pm		
2:30 pm		
3:00 pm		
3:30 pm		
4:00 pm		
4:30 pm		
5:00 pm		
5:30 pm		
6:00 pm		
6:30 pm		
7:00 pm		
7:30 pm		
8:00 pm		

8:30 pm		
9:00 pm		
9:30 pm		
10:00 pm		
10:30 pm		
11:00 pm		
11:30 pm		
12:00 am		

DAY SEVEN

Time	Planned Activity	What I actually did...
Example	**Work out**	**Went to a party**
5:00 am		
5:30 am		
6:00 am		
6:30 am		
7:00 am		
7:30 am		
8:00 am		
8:30 am		
9:00 am		
9:30 am		
10:00 am		
10:30 am		
11:00 am		
11:30 am		
12:00 noon		
12:30 pm		
1:00 pm		
2:00 pm		
2:30 pm		
3:00 pm		
3:30 pm		
4:00 pm		
4:30 pm		
5:00 pm		
5:30 pm		
6:00 pm		
6:30 pm		
7:00 pm		
7:30 pm		
8:00 pm		

8:30 pm		
9:00 pm		
9:30 pm		
10:00 pm		
10:30 pm		
11:00 pm		
11:30 pm		
12:00 am		

Discover

(Preparation) – "Action Plan Developed"

This portion is all about discovery. Discovering the root of the problems you're having with your health and why you haven't achieved your goals. Once you know and understand the root of the problem your journey to a new lifestyle will be easy.

On the following blank page write down these categories:

- Eating preferenes?

- Lifestyle?

- Goals?

Eating preferences:

1. What foods do you like or dislike?

2. What foods do you currently eat?

3. What foods do you want to eat?

4. What are your food preferences, (vegan? Paleo?)

Lifestyle:

1. What is your budget?

2. How many people are you cooking for?

3. Do you prefer to prepare meals in advance or a meal at a time?

4. Your cultural preferences?

Goals:

1. Are you looking to lose weight with healthy eating?

2. Are you looking to increase overall energy levels?

3. What are your specific health conditions?

PREPARATION NOTES:

Now its time to develop your plan.

When thinking about planning your meals, remember your A, B, C's – Awareness, Balance and Control. These are the building blocks of life-long, healthy eating habits that will help instill good habits

A = AWARENESS

Be aware of what you are eating and its nutritional value. What amounts of calories, fat and carbohydrates are in the foods you eat? Read labels and become food-conscious to make healthy eating decisions.

It is also important to look at all the foods and ingredients you are eating rather than focus on just one.

If not, you may inadvertently limit your access to quality foods and drinks. For instance, high fructose corn syrup is often mislabeled as "bad," even though there is no credible scientific evidence to support this claim. Instead, look at all of the combined sugars in your diet and make healthy decisions accordingly.

B = BALANCE

Balance your daily food selection to include whole-grain products, fruit, vegetables, dairy products and foods high in protein. You need more than 40 different nutrients for good health, and no single food supplies them all.
Offering balanced choices at every meal provides necessary nutrients for proper growth and health.

C = CONTROL

Control portion size and intake of foods high in fat, salt or sugar. Eat them in moderation and choose other foods to provide the balance and variety that are vital to good health.

Preparation for eating simple on a budget

1. Buy Whole Foods. Unprocessed foods are cheaper and more nutritious than processed foods. They also give you total control over the ingredients. Avoid anything that comes from a box 90% of the time. Proteins. Ground beef, frozen chicken breast, tuna cans, calves' liver, cottage cheese, plain yogurt, eggs, milk, whey, … Carbs. Pasta, rice, oats, potatoes, beans, apples, bananas, raisins, broccoli, spinach, cabbage, … Fats. Olive oil, fish oil, flax seeds, real butter, mixed nuts, …

2. Buy Cheap Proteins. You need 1g protein per pound of body-weight per day to build and

maintain muscle. Eating whole protein with each meal also helps fat loss as protein has a higher thermionic effect than other foods. Keep the steaks & salmon for special occasions. Buy eggs, milk, whey, mackerel, tuna, calves liver, frozen chicken breast, cottage cheese.

3.Buy Frozen Fruits & Veggies. Unfreeze berries in microwave and eat warm with cottage cheese. Put frozen spinach in a colander the night before and try one of these recipes the next day. Try also frozen beans & broccoli. Benefits: Save Money. Often half the price of fresh. Almost infinite shelf life when kept in freezer. And you can buy in bulk to get more discount. Save Time. Frozen fruits & veggies are per-washed and per-cut, which saves preparation time. Time is money. Nutrient Dense. If frozen right when picked, frozen fruits & veggies can contain more nutrients than fresh ones.

4. Buy Generic Food. And store brands. Raw foods like rice, pasta, eggs, milk, cottage cheese, frozen fruits/veggies, … taste like brand name foods once you get used to them. But they'll save you money on packaging & advertising.

5. Buy In Season Fruits & Veggies. Food grown in season tastes better and is cheaper. Root vegetables in the Winter. Apples & squash in the Fall. Broccoli & berries in the Summer. Buy Calorie Dense Foods. Whole milk, potatoes, rice, pasta & oats are filling, healthy and easy to stockpile. They'll help you get your daily caloric needs fast & cheap, and make gaining weight for skinny guys easier.

6. Buy From Local Farmers. Or farmer's markets. They aren't always cheaper, but you get tastier & better quality food and they often give you free stuff when you buy a lot. Find local farmers in your area here & here.

7. Drink Tap Water. Get a Britain pitcher and filter your tap water. It's cheaper than bottled water, soda or orange juice. One $8 filter cleans 40 gallons water and makes it taste a lot better.

8. Stop Buying Food Outside. Preparing your own food gives you total control over the ingredients and is cheaper than buying food at work/school. Take Food with You. Food containers for work/school, protein shake for the gym, bag of nuts when you go to the movies, … Eat Before Leaving Home. Eat breakfast, eat before doing the grocery, eat before going out with friends/family, …

9. Prepare Your Own Food. Cook all your meals for the day on waking up or before going to bed. It takes 30-40mins, saves you stress about what you'll be eating the rest of the day and you eat healthy while saving money. Stop Buying Processed Food. Buy oats instead of cereals, make home made protein bars, home made tomato sauce, home made pizza, … Keep it Simple. Make double portions, take leftovers with you, use cans of tuna & mackerel, rice & pasta, frozen veggies, … Learn to Cook from Scratch. Learn to work with spices & herbs. Invest in a good cook book.

10. Grow Your Own Food. Cheaper than frozen, tastes better and you control what you put on them to keep bugs off. Plant your own trees that grow berries, walnuts & apples. Buy chickens for free eggs & meat. More ideas: Square-Foot Gardening. Build a raised bed and divide it into sections of 1 square foot. Check Mel Bartholomew's site & book for how ti's. Container Gardening. Grow vegetables in containers on your balcony or doorstep. Check this & this guides. Rent Garden Plots. If you don't have a yard, some cities rent garden plots. Just Google rent garden plots in your state.

Conscious consuming
Most of the products and services we use in industrialized societies today are disposable, hazardous, and often, unnecessary. Yet our capitalist economy depends on our consumption of such products and services, and we are told that it's UN-American to question our role in this arrangement. Conscious Consumers dare to question; a whole host of variables might go into our decision-making, but the important thing is that we do that thinking.

Before We buy, we wonder:
Is this item in line with my values?
Does this product or service support my vision for a sustainable, equitable society?
Is there another product of service that is better aligned with my values?

5 values of conscious consuming:

1. health and safety conscious seek natural, organic and unmodified products that meet their essential health and nutrition needs. Avoid chemicals or pesticides that can harm your health or the planet. Look for standards and safeguards to ensure the quality of the products they consume.

2. Honesty conscious consumers insist that companies reliably and accurately detail product features and benefits. You will reward companies that are honest about processes and practices, authentic about products and accountable for their impact on the environment and larger society making unsubstantiated green claims or over promising benefits risks breeding cynicism and distrust.

3. Convenience faced with increasing constraints on your time and household budgets, conscious consumers are practical about purchasing decisions, balancing price with needs and desires and demanding quality. These consumers want to do whats easy, whats essential for getting by and making decisions that fit your lifestyles and budget.

4. Relationships who made it? Where does it come from? Am I getting back what I put into it? You want to find meaningful relationships with the brands in your life. Seek out opportunities to support the local economy when given the change, want to know the source of the products by and desire more personal interactions when doing business.

5. Doing good finally conscious consumers are concerned about the world and want to do their part to make it a better place. From seeking out environmentally friendly products to rewarding companies fair trade a labor practices you make choices that can help others. You want to make a difference, an want brands to do the same.

Eating Clean

The soul of clean eating is consuming food in its most natural state, or as close to it as possible. It is not a diet; it's a lifestyle approach to food and its preparation, leading to an improved life – one meal at a time.

- Eat five to six times a day. Three meals and two to three small snacks. Include a lean protein, plenty of fresh fruit and vegetables, and a complex carbohydrate with each meal. This keeps your body energized and burning calories efficiently all day long.
- Drink at least two liters of water a day
  Preferably from a reusable canteen, not plastic; we're friends of the environment here! Limit your alcohol intake to one glass of antioxidant-rich red wine a day.
- Get label savvy
  Clean foods contain just one or two ingredients. Any product with a long ingredient list is human-made and not considered clean.
- Avoid processed and refined foods
  This includes white flour, sugar, bread and pasta. Enjoy complex carbs such as whole grains instead.
- Know thy enemies
  Steer clear of anything high in saturated and trans fats, anything fried or anything high in sugar.
- Shop with a conscience
- Consume humanely raised and local meats. (lean meats such as turkey, fish, poultry)
- Choose organic whenever possible
  If your budget limits you, make meat, eggs, dairy and the dirty dozen if our organic priorities.
- Consume healthy fats. Try to have essential fatty acids, or Eras, every day.
- Watch your portions
- Reduce your carbon footprint. Eat produce that is seasonal and local. It is less taxing on your wallet and our environment.
- Slow down and savor – mindful-eating. Never rush through a meal. Food tastes best when savored. Enjoy every bite!
- Take it to go. Meal preparation. Pack a cooler for work or outings so you always have clean eats on the go.

Meal preparation

Planning your meals for the week is essential if you have a busy schedule, and it helps you stay on track of your meals. A quick easy grab and go.

Before beginning any meal prep, it is recommended that you have various food storage containers on hand, you are going to need them!

The Two P's - Plan and Prep

HOW TO:

-Pick one day a week as your "plan and prep" day

- Grocery shop on this day as well!

PLAN

1. Plan your meals for the week out using the following guideline:

- Protein + Starch + Vegetable (and be making sure to get your healthy fats in!)

- Protein options that I recommend: I have put a * next to my favorites!

-Chicken Breasts* Boneless, Skinless

-Chicken thighs are okay for specific recipes

-Ground Beef – 85% lean or higher

-Ground Turkey* – 93% lean or higher*

-Fish – Salmon,* Tilapia, Shrimp*

-Eggs (hard boil a bunch for the week!)

-Steak, Pork, or Sausage are all options too, but I don't eat those meats enough to offer advice on how to best prepare them for meal prep!

Vegetarian or Vegan?

Try plant based proteins:

beans (black beans, garbanzo beans, kidney beans, etc.) edamame, tofu, tempeh !

Starch options: opt for whole grain, complex carbohydrates as your fuel!

- Quinoa— you can add whatever flavors/spices of dish to quinoa to boost flavor

- Sweet potato

- Brown rice

- Pasta

- Potato

- Rice Varities: Jasmine*, Basmati*, Wild Grain, Etc.

- Buckwheat

- Amaranth

(there are other options as well this is just a basic list)

Vegetable options: leafy greens are your best bet here! I have put a * next to my favorites!

- Spinach
- Green Beans
- Mushrooms
- Asparagus
- Brocoli
- Cucumber
- Red, Yellow, Orange Peppers
- Zucchini
- Kale
- Bok Choy
- Spaghetti Squash (unsure if this is even considered a vegetable)
- Carrots
- Tomatoes
- Sugar Snap Peas

2. Check to make sure you have **all** the ingredients for all recipes before hand!
3. Add necessary items to the shopping list

PREP

1. Grocery shop for the week
2. Peel, chop, cut all raw veggies for the week to put in lunch or to have as a snack
(Healthy choices are easier to make when they're ready to be eaten!)
3. Repeat the process for any fruit that requires cutting to be eaten
4. Prep your protein/meals (see below)
-Make specific meals to eat as alternating left overs
-Make items to store in the freezer and eat at a later time

Make your meat "basic" to be used in a variety of ways through out the week
Now, you can take prepping as far as you want to.
You can:
1. Cook enough protein, veggies, starches to eat for the week
(keeping these items basic will make them more versatile to use during the week)
OR
2.Cook two meals to generate enough meals to alternate for the week (five days of dinners)

MEAT PREP

Preparing

- Make ground beef/ ground turkey meatballs and freeze for a later date
- Make homemade burgers for now and to freeze for a later date
- Crockpot freezer meals, google this! I am not at that level of prepping

Cooking - cook as much of your protein that you would like to have for the week
- Grill chicken in bulk with a variety of seasonings to switch up the flavor during the week
- Bake chicken in bulk
- Use your crockpot! Makes enough of a dish to have for the week!
- Cook chicken in chicken broth in the crockpot and use as shredded chicken to add to recipes for the week (think crokpot chicken tacos, to put on top of salad)
- Sauté ground beef/ground turkey with a little bit of garlic powder
(eat as is through out the week or create dishes with it such as tacos, beef and peppers, etc.)
- Hard boil enough eggs for the week as a lunch option or go to protein based snack

TIMING IS EVERYTHING

Do you know the best times to eat certain foods?

Banana:

Eat at lunch – strengthens immune system and improves skin

Do no eat at dinner – may lead to mucus formation and disturb digestion

Orange:

Eat at snack – improves digestion, increases metabolism

Do not eat breakfast – eating on empty stomach may cause stomach irritation and gastritis

Apple:

Eat at breakfast – apple contains pectin which lowers blood sugar and cholesterol levels

Do not eat at dinner – pectin is hard to digest at night, increase stomach acid

Tomato:

Eat at breakfast – improves digestion, increase metabolism

Do not eat at dinner- pectin and oxalic acid in tomatoes may cause stomach swelling if eaten for dinner

Meat:

Eat at lunch – great source of iron, reduces fatigue and vulnerability to disease

Do not eat at dinner – takes around 4-6 hours to digest, can damage digestive system

Rice:

Eat at lunch – high in carbohydrate, gives energy for the whole day

Do not eat at dinner – leads t weight gain

Potato:

Eat at breakfast – potato starch lowers cholesterol, rich in minerals

Do not eat at Dinner – much higher in calories compared to other vegetables, may lead to weight gain if eaten at dinner

Nuts:

Eat at lunch – lowers risk of blood pressure and keeps heart healthy

Do not eat at dinner – high in fat and calories, so eating at dinner may lead to weight gain

Yogurt:

Eat at dinner – helps in faster digestion of dinner, curbs late night snack craving

Do not eat at breakfast – makes the empty stomach very acidic and has the potential to damage the stomach lining

Dark chocolate:

Eat at breakfast – provides anti oxidants which reduce aging and risk of heart disease

Do not eat at snack – snack time dark chocolates are dangerous as body fat increases

Eating with seasons

Seasonal food is fresher and so tends to be tastier and more nutritious. You get to reconnect with nature's cycles and the passing of time. Eat in natures rhythm, everything in the universe has its place, things are what they are for reason. Your produce is consumed at its most nutritious point. The nutrients in your produce diminish drastically after being picked. For an example strawberries that you purchase from Africa in the winter season may be already a few week old. By that time most of the nutritional value of the strawberries have been lost.

You will feel better and increase good health in the changing seasons. Which is why in today's society its hard for our bodies to adjust to changing seasons. In cold months you want to eat spicy foods warm foods, in the hot months you want to eat foods that are cooling and raw. This is how nature intended it. If you eat in season, you will naturally be eating the right foods to keep your system in balance.

Eating fruits in the spring will clean the colon. Eating ripe melon will cleanse the kidneys. When you eat with the season it prepares your body for the upcoming season. You want to cleanse your colon before you cleanse the kidney. By doing so, this will prepare your body for the fall and winter when we eat grains and meats that help our body to keep warm. In other words mother nature created seasons for a reason and she knows her stuff.

Fall foods:
apples, beets, brussel sprouts, cranberries, figs, winter squash, swiss chard

Winter foods:
radishes, grapefruit, kale, leeks, lemons, oranges, chestnuts

Spring foods:
Avocados, cherries, mangos, spinach, strawberries, apricots, asparagus

Summer foods:
blueberries, bell peppers, corn, cucumbers, pineapple, watermelon, broccoli

Best times to eat

- *Breakfast:* ideal time 7:00 am – 8:00 am
  don't have it later than 10:00 am, remember to eat within at least 30 minutes of waking up

- *Lunch:* ideal time 12:30 pm – 2:00 pm
  don't have it later than 4:00 pm, remember an ideal time gap between breakfast and lunch is 4 hours

- *Dinner:* ideal time 6:00 pm – 9:00 pm
  don't have it later than 10:00 pm, remember the meal should be at least 3 hours before sleep

PORTIONS FOR BALANCED MEALS

Breakfast	Contain a diary, fruits, grains and protein
Snack	Contain diary and fruits
Lunch	Contain fruit, protein, grains, and vegetables
Snack	Contain diary and Vegetables
Dinner	Contain vegetables, protein, and grains

HEALTHY SHOPPING LIST CHART

Fresh Fruit	bananas apples oranges grapes pears Asian pears strawberries blueberries avocado olives lemons
Greens and Veggies	leafy greens spinach kale tomatoes bell peppers cucumbers celery purple cabbage
Frozen Section non GMO	mixed vegetables corn edamame peas black eyed peas chickpeas baby lima beans
Whole Grains	thick rolled oats steel cut oats wheat berries brown rice quinoa whole grain flour whole grain bread whole grain bread
Bulk, Nuts, and Seeds	almonds cashews pistachios hazelnuts walnuts pecans hemp seeds, flaxseeds, chia seeds fresh almond butter

Dried Fruit	Dates Cranberries Raisins
Sweeteners	pure maple syrup Maple sugar local raw honey unsweetened coconut flakes
Beans and Legumes	black beans lentils
Tubers/Roots and Vegetables	potatoes sweet potatoes carrots
Fats	coconut oil olive oil avocado oil
Non diary milk	flax milk (optional) yogurt (optional) almond milk (optional) Soy milk (optional)
Animal Products	wild seafood turkey chicken pasture raised eggs grassfed beef

Now that we have developed an action plan lets, start documenting. Here is a meal chart to record meals for the week.

	BREAKFAST	LUNCH	DINNER
MONDAY			
TUESDAY			
WEDNESDAY			
THURSDAY			
FRIDAY			
SATURDAY			
SUNDAY			

Reset

(Action) - "Behavior reinforced"

The 4ᵗʰ week is about resetting your body and giving you that extra push to get back on a healthy track. Detoxing helps rid the body of hard to digest and blood sugar spiking foods. Think of a detox as a reset button. You are reinforcing good eating habits by reminding your body how it feels when its fed healthy foods and is well hydrated. After this reset you will be eager to eat healthy again.

Rather than following an extreme detox plan that limits just about every food except fruit and veg while at the same time getting you to down a nasty 'detox' drink every day, this plan is safer and more sensible and shouldn't leave you short on nutrients if you follow it for just one week.

WHY IS WATER DETOX SO IMPORTANT?
Water is, quite literally, the river on which our good health flows. Water carries nutrients to our cells, aids digestion by forming stomach secretions, flushes our bodies of wastes, and keeps our kidneys healthy. It keeps our moisture-rich organs (our skin, eyes, mouth, and nose) functioning well, it lubricates and cushions our joints, and it regulates our body temperature and our metabolism, just to name a few of its many functions.

Water also plays a crucial role in disease prevention. Without enough water flowing through our systems to carry out wastes and toxins, we would literally drown in our own poisonous metabolic wastes.

Consult your doctor before beginning any detoxification program. Best results incorporate physical activity.

Foods to include in the plan

Your plan can include:

•Fruit– your plan can include any fruit including fresh, frozen, dried or canned in natural fruit juice. This includes apples, bananas, pears, oranges, grapefruit, satsumas, sultanas, raisins, pineapple, mango, kiwi fruit, strawberries, raspberries, blackcurrants, nectarines, peaches, melons, star fruit etc

•Fruit juice– either make homemade fruit juices or smoothies from fresh fruit, or drink ready-made juices. Make sure ready-made juices are labelled as being 'pure' or 'unsweetened'.

•Vegetables– eat any vegetables including fresh, frozen or canned in water (without salt added). This includes carrots, onions, turnip, swede, sprouts, cabbage, peppers, mushrooms, sweetcorn, peppers, leeks, courgettes, broccoli, cauliflower, salad, tomatoes, cucumber, spring onions etc

•Beans and lentils– eat any beans, including those that have been dried or canned in water. This includes red kidney, haricot, cannellini, butter, black eye, pinto, red lentils, green lentils and brown lentils

•Tofu and Quorn

•Oats– sprinkle oats over fresh fruit or use to make porridge, sweetened with honey and fresh fruit

•Potatoes– all types

•Brown rice and rice noodles

•Rye crackers, rice cakes and oatcakes

•Fresh fish– eat any fresh fish including cod, plaice, mackerel, salmon, lobster, crab, trout, haddock, tuna, prawns, Dover sole, red mullet, halibut, lemon sole, monkfish, swordfish etc. Canned fish in water is suitable too eg salmon or tuna

•Unsalted nut– eat any including Brazil, peanuts, almonds, cashew, hazel nuts, macadamia, pecans, pine nuts, pistachio, walnuts etc

•Unsalted seeds– eat any including sunflower and pumpkin

•Plain popcorn– without sugar or salt

•Live natural yogurt

•Extra virgin olive oil and balsamic vinegar

•Garlic, ginger and fresh herbs

•Ground black pepper

•Honey

•Water– at least 2 liters a day. Tap or mineral water is fine.

•Herbal or fruit teas

Foods to avoid during your detox

•Red meat, chicken, turkey and any meat products like sausages, burgers, and pate

•Milk, cheese, eggs, cream

•Butter and margarine

•Any food that contains wheat including bread, croissants, cereals, cakes, biscuits, pies, pastry, quiche, battered or breadcrumbed foods, etc

•Crisps and savoury snacks including salted nuts

•Chocolate, sweets, jam and sugar

•Processed foods, ready meals, ready-made sauces and takeaways

•Alcohol

•Coffee and tea

•Sauces, pickles, shop bought salad dressing, mayonnaise

•Salt
•Fizzy drinks and squashes, including diet versions

STEP 1= Add water
STEP 2 =Add fruit
STEP 3 =Let water infuse (5 minute minimum)
STEP 4 =Drink about half your body weight in water or a gallon a day.

<u>DAY 1:</u>
Cucumbers, Strawberries and Basil - Boots immune system

<u>Day 2:</u>
Cucumbers, Strawberries, Lemons, and Oranges - Helps boost energy

<u>Day 3:</u>
Apples and Cinnamon Sticks - Removes heavy metals from your system

<u>Day 4:</u>
Lemons and Raspberries - Fight inflammation

<u>Day 5:</u>
Green apples, Cucumbers and Mint - Helps weight loss

<u>Day 6:</u>
Strawberries, Cucumbers, Lime, and Mint - Relieves stress

<u>Day 7:</u>
Cucumbers, Limes, Lemons, Grapefruit, and Mint - Lowers blood pressure

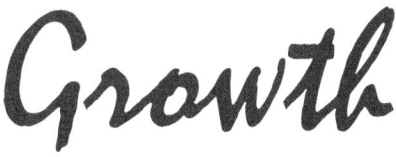

Growth

(Maintenance) - "Self-Efficacy"

The section is week 5, week 5 is about growth. Growth the act or process, or a manner of growing; development; gradual increase.

This week look at how much you've grown and learned so far. Take time to reflect on your results. Have you found meaning in eating again? Do you see the purpose of food more important than you did before?

Take this time to analyze the changes, the habits broken, and the connection you have made with eating. Write it down and remember to continue these habits. Reflective practice is, in its simplest form, thinking about or reflecting on what you do. It is closely linked to the concept of learning from experience, in that you think about what you did, and what happened, and decide from that what would you do differently next time. Once you can self reflect on your lifestyle change journey you will continue to grow, maintain, make better eating choices, eat simple, and with a purpose.

Reflection:

_____

_____

_____

_____

_____

_____

time to restart

Going back to the basics strengthens your foundation of healthy eating.

I will eat mindfully, be more aware of each bite I take

Pace not to race eat slowly and with intention

When I eat, just eat without distraction

Calm Without calories, find true comfort and soothing without food-conscious

Eat less, nourish more. Eat foods that nurture my body